Clinics in Human Lactation

Mentoring Our Future

By Denise Altman RN, IBCLC, LCCE

Mentoring Our Future

Denise Altman RN, IBCLC, LCCE

Praeclarus Press, LLC

2504 Sweetgum Lane

Amarillo, Texas 79124 USA

806-367-9950

www.PraeclarusPress.com

DISCLAIMER

The information contained in this publication is advisory only and is not intended to replace sound clinical judgment or individualized patient care. The author disclaims all warranties, whether expressed or implied, including any warranty as the quality, accuracy, safety, or suitability of this information for any particular purpose.

ISBN: 978-1-939807-81-6

For my mom, the perfect lady who always makes anyone feel at ease;

And for my dad, my first and longest business mentor.

And again, for Jim, who makes it easier on me when I say "yes" to too many projects.

Table of Contents

Introduction

The book began as a conversation in a restaurant.

I was attending a conference in Philadelphia and had presented a small business topic about diversifying revenue streams while managing costs, with mentoring as one example. During dinner that night, a physician seated at my table asked me to elaborate on what I was currently doing in my practice, then wanted my opinion on her own conundrum. She had a practice specializing in breastfeeding support, and she was getting calls from other doctors seeking help establishing their own program or just wanting additional breastfeeding support knowledge. She felt that this was a great potential revenue source for her business, particularly given the time investment she would need to make. However, she stated that doctors don't traditionally charge each other for training, and she felt ambivalent about going against tradition. We discussed possible approaches to get around the issue, but I felt that she probably left the restaurant still unsure about whether to proceed.

I left the restaurant thinking that medical schools–where the training is primarily done by doctors–charge quite a bit for the transfer of specialized knowledge.

I also started thinking about how we learn on an advanced level. Not just the book stuff, but the real, down-in-the-trenches knowledge that comes hard won and creates instincts and gut feelings for practice approach. Who teaches that to us, and who helps form who we are professionally? Of course it's a multitude of experiences and interactions, but if we are lucky, we encounter a mentor to help guide us along. If we are really lucky, we will have more than one.

Over the next couple of months, this conversation remained with me. Others who attended the conference emailed me with their own questions about mentoring others and creating programs. When preparing for the presentation, I had looked for resources about tapping into or creating a mentoring program, but nothing specific existed, so I drew on my experiences as a hospital clinical educator, as well as a private practice LC. I also used the business model for mentoring that I had incorporated for my work in both settings. As I got more questions from other LCs, I started looking for a description of the mentor lactation consultant-not what to teach-but rather the "who" and "why." Nothing.

This is my attempt to fill a void, or at least get the ball rolling.

In these pages, I have outlined what I believe are the nuts and bolts of mentoring, which is much more than just training. I began with research and outlined the basic structure for mentoring, but soon realized that I needed real life stories about good and bad mentoring experiences. I have included many personal stories from both leaders and worker bee's in our field; I dearly love listening to people tell me their tales. You will not find the name of one mentor who is held up as an example, although you will recognize some of the names behind the personal experiences. I want you, the reader, to be able to put yourself in the mentoring position, picturing yourself in that role rather than comparing yourself to someone you might perceive as impossible to live up to. I hope you read this and find yourself striving to grow in a new direction as a result.

The practice challenges that are included are also from real-life scenarios and are not intended to illustrate right or wrong answers. Instead, I hope they stimulate your thinking, even if you are unlikely to experience them in your own practice setting. Sometimes, a new and different problem can inspire creative thinking and solutions or even opportunities for your own worksite.

I intentionally did not include the "what to teach." This is constantly evolving and certainly isn't the same for all learners. Rather, I have tried to stay directed on the elements of mentoring and creating a mentoring program or process. I truly hope this book is a resource for anyone who wants to help others on the pathway to becoming professional lactation specialists at any level. I am writing to clinical nurse managers, WIC coordinators, small business owners, La Leche League Leaders, nurses, doctors, midwives, doulas, volunteers, or any breastfeeding advocate.

I really hope that you will email and tell me your successes as well as your challenges. I can be found at obrnmom@aol.com.

Mentoring Our Future

Guide- One who leads or directs another's way
Train- To make prepared (as by exercise) for a test of skill
Teach- a) To cause to know something; to cause to know
　　　b) To instruct by precept, example, or experience.
Mentor- a trusted counselor or guide

(Webster, 2010)

Each of these words, found in the online Webster's dictionary, offers a brief definition that can relate to the education of future breastfeeding advocates. However, only the definition for mentor states the human emotion connection. In the stories of mentoring that are found throughout this book, the emotional connection is emphasized by the storyteller in all. Truly defining a mentor and differentiating this from a teacher or trainer is very difficult because people have very different perceptions of this role. However, it seems as though the emotional connection is a very necessary part of the relationship.

Chapter 1. Historical Mentoring

Mentoring is the movement beyond the basic instructional knowledge into the practical application of knowledge through continued learning with interactive relationships. Currently, all categories of the medical profession begin with an academic baseline education. Individuals must first learn from books before they learn from patients. Clinical training and instruction is a necessary component for all healthcare-based professions because the book can only teach within limits.

When considering the traditional healthcare-focused professionals that may offer breastfeeding support, some that come to mind are midwives, doctors, and nurses. In the U.S. specifically, from the 1800s to early 1900s, students in any of these professions lived near—or even with their mentors. Their training was immersed within the activities of daily life, and all started with a foundation of the student performing basic tasks initially, with responsibilities building as the knowledge level and skills increased. This was often known as an apprenticeship. However, with the coming of the industrial age, mentoring evolved into a more formalized "teaching with training" concept that followed a standardized course of education. The practical or clinical aspects of learning were and are still heavily emphasized, but the individualized and/or one to one educating is greatly diminished.

The Profession of Lactation Consultants

Lactation Consultants have a relatively short professional history. Traditionally, birth and breastfeeding support through the ages was found primarily within the family and community, woman to woman. There has always been a need for supplementary or mother-replacement feedings due to illness or death, although it was definitely in the minority because substitutes for human milk were unsafe. Wet nursing, instead, was a far more accepted practice if the baby couldn't receive his own mother's milk. With industrialization and mass manufacturing, this slowly began to change. There is documented evidence that household advice books, even in the 1860s, encouraged early weaning due to the onset of prepared foods and cheaper glass bottles. One of the most famous advice books was "Mrs. Beeton's Book of Household Management". In it, the author stated that bottle feeding was "more nutritious" and even "that babies will be less liable to infectious disease"

(Flanders, 2004).

By the 1950s, breastfeeding initiation rates reached a reported all time low of 20-22%. This is generally considered due to women entering the workforce in large numbers during World War II, creating an increased need for commercial-grade artificial baby milk in mass quantities. The unexpected result was that breastfeeding was no longer considered desirable, healthy, or even normal.

October 17, 1956, was the date of the first meeting of a breastfeeding support group created by seven women, who began discussing the lack of breastfeeding knowledge and help while attending a church picnic. This group fast became an international resource for mother- to- mother support known as La Leche League. Leader applicants were, and are, mentored by an experienced Leader who followed very specific guidelines. The groups themselves rely on the interaction of all, rather than one expert providing all of the information; although the meetings follow prescribed topics and trained Leaders ensure that the information is accurate and breastfeeding specific. The experience and help often has a profound influence on women, and many times they can relate their experiences with LLL years later, even when becoming grandmothers.

A Personal Experience
Cindi Freeman IBCLC, LLLL
Private Practice Lactation Consultant

"She was a total stranger to me; twenty minutes of talking on the phone changed my life."

Cindi met her mentor over the phone when she reached out for help as a new mother. She was having painful feedings, but more importantly, difficulty coping with new motherhood. She can recall the basic topic of the conversation, but not the specifics. What is clear in her mind was how her mentor communicated in a relaxing tone of voice, matter of fact but encouraging. Her mentor suggested that Cindi attend a La Leche League meeting that week, then almost a year later after they had developed a deeper connection, she suggested that Cindi consider becoming a Leader.

While training as a Leader, Cindi got to know her mentor on a more personal level. Her children were older and leaving home; this allowed Cindi to see the results of the mothering styles that she promoted, as well as how she interacted, even with those closest to her. Cindi saw that for her Leader-Trainer there was no difference between the mentoring and the mothering; that the way she taught others had a parent nurturing quality without being overboard. Those that know Cindi describe her communication methods in very similar terms-particularly that Cindi is a whole hearted listener, with lots of positive reinforcement.

When trying to identify the connection with her mentor, Cindi states,

"It wasn't what she said, but how she said it. She could have said, "You should bring me the moon," and I would have said, "OK, sure." So I became a Leader and sat for the exam. I certainly never planned this course for my life. She inspires people, and changes their thinking. The field that she worked in is irrelevant; it was the way she connected with me and others. She is still doing it even today."

In 1982, La Leche League International, as an organization, began to recognize the importance of more formal support and partnered with UNICEF for a pilot program to train low-income women in Brazil as breastfeeding counselors. This led to peer counselor programs all over the world, and even provided the basis and structure for the development of the WIC peer counselor programs. They were also the driving force for the establishment of the International Board of Lactation Consultant Examiners, as well as the creation of the certification exam for professional breastfeeding specialists, administered for the first time in 1985.

Though the first Lactation Consultants were mostly La Leche League Leaders, LCs today come from a variety of different backgrounds; from doctors and nurses, to lawyers, singers, writers, engineers, public relations professionals, caterers, school teachers, chemists, nutritionists, even (at least one) professional ballerina--although there are still a big block of Leaders as well. Because of the diverse backgrounds and education, entry into the profession begins at multiple starting points, but the critical element, with increasing importance, is clinical training, particularly in the form of mentoring.

Chapter 2. Considerations for Mentoring

All of these historical accounts seem to be related, especially when looking at the evolution of professional breastfeeding support. The lactation profession has a strong medical focus and increasing recognition as a valid member of the healthcare team. This translates to more Lactation Consultants in titled, paid positions for large organizations, such as hospitals, WIC clinics, health departments, and even universities. The end users, the mother and her partner, are also starting to recognize the value of educated breastfeeding support and seek out care providers who offer this service when preparing for birth or when making other healthcare decisions.

The best measuring tool of the profession is the IBLCE exam, which incorporates a variety of testing methods to identify strengths, weaknesses, and baseline competency. As a result of consumer demand, IBCLC candidate applications increased by 25% from 2008 to 2009 (IBLCE, 2010); growth that would make any business corporation ecstatic. At this rapid growth rate, standardizing education and training has been extremely difficult, if not impossible. Exam candidates must meet minimum education requirements, but the majority of their knowledge must be from hands on, patient interaction. In order to obtain this, the learner must be partnered with an experienced teacher, not only to protect the patient, but also to ensure effective learning and skills accumulation.

"Mentoring provides important personal guidance for the development of a new generation of mother-baby supporters. It is a hallmark of our profession that we have learned from those that have come before us. Now we have a more systemic approach that allows the public to be assured that the IBCLC has superior knowledge."

Elizabeth Brooks JD, IBCLC
Board of Directors/International Lactation Consultants Association

The IBLCE is not the only organization to require practical experience before process completion; most organizations with programs directed toward patient care or mother support also have this requirement. Related examples are The WIC Peer Counselor Program and La Leche League. The personal knowledge regarding evidence-based practice can be gained from books, journals, websites, and class instructors. In fact, formal classes with an established curriculum are the most recognized way to gain a solid foundation of baseline knowledge. The setting can be an academic classroom, conference, or even online. Regardless of the setting, the instructor or teacher of the course functions as a guide to identify and direct learning needs within the curriculum or framework.

Once the baseline knowledge is established, the learner must then build on it with practical application, and continued, perhaps less formal, coursework or instruction. In fact, many times the learner doesn't realize how much they don't know until confronted with real-life scenarios for application. Ultimately, there isn't a substitute for practical and clinical application of knowledge and theory. Practical application moves beyond the classroom or structured framework, involving real people with unanticipated problems or concerns. This is often where the teacher becomes the mentor, although this role is not necessarily completed by the same or even one individual.

This explains how the student benefits from the mentoring relationship. But what's in it for the mentor? In other words, why would someone want to become a mentor? There are several possible reasons, and they are usually personalized to the individual who is considering mentoring.

Strengthening the Profession

Because the practice of lactation support is such a young profession, leaders and learners are experiencing a continuing evolution toward standardized training and education. Without consistency, it is very difficult to create a measuring tool for competency and therefore gain continuing and increasing recognition as team members. How and what to teach others has been a question since the very beginning.

A Personal Story
Jeanne Rago BA, IBCLC, FILCA
Private Practice Lactation Consultant

Jeanne Rago was among the first La Leche League Leaders to take the first board exam, and then begin practice in the new profession of Lactation. She writes,

"The concept of mentoring made me think about what we, as fledgling LCs, were told would lay the groundwork for credibility in our new field. In a word, it was professionalism. Our professionalism must be the thread that ran through all that we did, wrote, spoke. I took this very seriously, as my personal ethical contribution to my beloved work, my responsibility as one of the frightened first to set out in our new field. I had the sense that we were all moving out and forward from this central point of understanding that we were laying the groundwork, we must be above reproach in all that we did. It was required of whatever we would submit to our Journal of Human Lactation, *then a slim booklet of personal exchanges about our work and our questions of one another. We mentored one another that way.*

My vision of professionalism, however, evolved from the desire to provide genuine dedication and caring for a mother in need of my expertise: I simply having traversed that road before her. The person who put me on this journey was my own mother who modeled so much to me and taught me to reach out for help when something was important to me, and I was in some struggle alone. The Mother Mentor sent me to the La Leche League Mentors (Leaders) who walked with me during those early days of loving my baby through breastfeeding. Their voices, their words and patience imprinted a memory of kindness so deep that it helps me hear myself in each mother who calls for help. Mentoring.

My father mentored me through some social awkwardness by telling me to just say "thank you" when I received a compliment instead of fidgeting and mumbling awkwardly. He said it helped the person giving the compliment to feel good about their gesture. This mentoring taught me to receive and give back all at once. He also showed me how to shake hands with someone. To this day, I greet each new client, hearing my mother tell me to stand up straight and look a person in the eyes, offering a smile at the pleasure of meeting them. I realize now that the "firm, but not crushing" handshake that my father made me practice with him has given me a sense of confidence in myself and, I hope, inspires confidence in me by a mother who wants so much to trust me to help her.

There is an evolution and a polishing of a persona, an individual style that comes from loving guidance, shared goals, and hard work. The outcome of positive mentoring is a gift to the mentor, the mentored, and all the people whose lives they touch. Mentoring well reaches forward and touches the future."

A solid foundation, measurable competency, and a standardized education process can have an economic impact as well. Today, the drive for reimbursement by insurance companies to pay for professional lactation support is the goal of many LC leaders in the United States. Many believe that as the numbers of professional breastfeeding specialists grow, consumer demand will pressure insurers to change their policies of no or sporadic coverage for consult fees. The consumers themselves will create the demand as they personally experience the benefits of knowledgeable professional support.

Personal Growth

Mentoring others can lead to personal growth, emotionally and intellectually. Lactation knowledge resembles a flowing river fed by small streams. No one person has a knowledge base made up exclusively of personal and clinical experience. For example, research begins with a simple conversation about an experience, leading to an idea, the creation of a process, implementation, translation of results, and finally information distributed to others in a variety of outlets and mechanisms. When a lactation consultant has a difficult case, often the first thing she does is consult message board archives, peers, or other personal resources for feedback and suggestions. Knowledge is meant to be shared in order to increase.

"I love being a clinical mentor because I get to learn and stretch and grow along with my interns. In order to teach clinical reasoning, I have to examine my strategies, evaluate them in light of recent evidence, and think them out clearly enough to put them into words."

Cathy Watson Genna BS, IBCLC
Author, Researcher, Speaker

Those who mentor others often report a sense of energy and personal growth, either during and/or after the relationship. It can be very rewarding when a learner recognizes your personal strengths and wisdom gained by experience. Everyone needs positive reinforcement, and a learner who is excited about what she is doing provides that to her mentor through the working relationship, but also in the form of verbal feedback. Their excitement and new-found passion is a renewal that transfers to the mentor as well.

Mentoring is a great way to ensure that skills remain current, not to mention valid. Like learners, many mentors begin to realize their own knowledge deficits once they begin to teach others. This is very normal, and even desirable. Lactation is an ever-changing field with new research and techniques emerging at a rapid pace. It can be very easy to get focused on the demands of the workplace and forget that education is an ongoing process at every level. Individuals who remain static in their practice, "this is the way we do it," may not be practicing evidence-based care and are probably not assisting their patients in the best way possible. Sometimes, just the questions that emerge when training a newcomer allow a seasoned expert a greater realization of her own learning opportunities.

Mentoring also allows the teacher to rediscover her passion in her practice. When detailing their reasons for entering the field, most Lactation Consultants report having some personal connection with breastfeeding, although not necessarily within their own mother-baby experience. This can erode over time, particularly for individuals experiencing overload or early signs of burnout. Teaching others can renew that sense of personal connection. Mentoring can allow the LC to see mothers and babies experiencing what once seemed to be the same old problems in a whole new light. The sense of satisfaction received during consults and helping families that may have diminished over a long period of time can be renewed as a result of mentoring.

A Personal Story
Linda Smith, IBCLC
Professional Educator, Author

Linda Smith is considered one of the "mothers" of lactation. Her first professional roots were in coaching as a physical education teacher in schools; these roots are still very much a part of her work. As a La Leche League Leader, she was instrumental (with others) in forming lactation consulting into a profession.

However, there was a point in time where she was seriously close to burnout and questioning whether or not she was truly making a difference. She writes,

"I found myself getting angry and frustrated when "this" mother has the same problems as the last ten or twenty. Didn't she hear what I told the others?!

Of course she didn't because she couldn't. So I turned my attention to teaching and writing-changing the healthcare system and its providers.

Put it in another way, I got very good at pulling mothers out of the river. However, something or someone was still throwing them into the river upstream. I set about trying to do what I could to prevent the problems in the first place, rather than fixing problems after they occurred. Besides, I figured out that teaching one doctor or ten nurses got me more bang for my buck than helping 100 more women."

Finding a new direction helped her regain her passion and focus. Mentoring and teaching others allows Linda to use her strengths, knowledge, and experience in a more personally satisfying way.

Costs of Mentoring

The decision to mentor can be a difficult one because mentoring is not without costs of all types. Mentoring can be time consuming, takes patience, and even contains some element of risk as the trainee begins to practice with indirect supervision. Although the benefits are potentially great, no individual should make the decision to mentor or create a program without also weighing all considerations, including some that may be negative.

Training and mentoring comes with a significant financial cost, whether it's with an individual or within an organization. Many professions, especially business and industry, know to the penny the cost of training or replacing an employee. Unfortunately, given the newness of the lactation profession, the broad salary range, and the varied roles of the lactation consultant, it is difficult to even ballpark the expense of teaching and training-at least beyond books and classes. Even established internship programs through hospitals contain a heavy cost center, particularly since there is usually more than one trainee. Because it is absorbed within a big organization, the perception is often that training costs are minimal, or even free which can create frustration for managers trying to meet budget and productivity requirements.

Productivity is primarily considered to be time spent on patient care, but it can also include preparing for classes, reporting, networking, or any other duties of the lactation consultant. For the mentor, productivity is cut almost in half on average, particularly at the beginning of a mentoring relationship. For example, an inpatient LC (ILC) may spend an average of 30 minutes at the bedside helping a new mother with latch. If the ILC is training a new intern as well, that time can be extended by an additional 20 to 30 minutes. Even if the intern is close to completing her training, the ILC will need to spend about 10-15 minutes following up with the new mother to ensure patient satisfaction and adequate support, as well as spending additional time reviewing and signing off on documentation by the learner.

Often instruction and support go beyond traditional work hours. Therefore, while the mentor is working for a salary in an organization, there is a personal cost to even the most organized person. Many mentors will spend significant time on the phone with their trainee after hours. Or at the very least, they will find themselves mentally reviewing training issues, difficult consults, or even preparing for the next learning session during "off hours."

Mentoring is fatiguing because there is both a physical and an emotional component. When a job is well learned, the worker can subconsciously create mental down time, such as spending less energy on patients who primarily need only positive reinforcement or taking a full lunch break during a low census. When mentoring, this is generally not an option because the learner always has questions and the mentor is continuously on the lookout for teaching opportunities. As the mentorship nears completion, the learner may actually experience an increased need for support, as she realizes that her training is almost at and end and she will be soloing without the safety net of her mentor.

Because of these factors, individuals who already have a heavy workload or multiple responsibilities need to take a hard look at how mentoring others will fit into existing tasks. There are many options that can be utilized to stabilize and balance established responsibilities, but they need to be in place before the training relationship ever begins.

Program coordinators or mentors should evaluate clock hours needed to establish clinical skills, as well as time spent creating, implementing, and evaluating a training program. If productivity is measured in consult hours or patient visits, organizational administrators need to be included in decision making as well. Individuals who are self-employed need to consider time away from business concerns as a productivity cost, since the customer base must be continuously renewed and marketing is an ongoing time need. While cost alone should not be a factor to refuse mentoring, it definitely should be considered during decision making, but can often be overlooked.

Chapter 3. Being the Mentor

There are many terms for mentoring: teacher, trainer, coach, team leader, supervisor, and so on. Many trainers approach their role as a necessary evil, for example, a worker in a large organization who is required to assist with new employee training-whether he wants to or not. This can actually create more harm than good. If an individual in a new role encounters a trainer who is indifferent or worse, resentful of this responsibility, then the learning opportunity will be diminished or ruined all together. Even worse, the new hire may decide to seek employment elsewhere, wasting all of the financial and physical resources and requiring the hiring process to be restarted from square one.

Instead, mentoring and training should be done by those truly interested in the roles. Mentoring is a heavy responsibility and implies a long term connection between the mentor and learner. A good mentor should be generous with her knowledge; practice within evidence-based guidelines, while knowing the rationale and purpose; have patience; be an effective communicator; and, most important, have a good sense of humor. Mentoring takes a large amount of time, both with and away from the learner, and a good mentor is always learning themselves. Therefore, a good mentor should invest in their own learning by joining at least one professional organization, reviewing current research, being an active community partner, and attending conferences regularly.

A Personal Experience
Ann Conlon-Smith, IBCLC
Pediatric Office Lactation Consultant

Ann Conlon-Smith can point to two women who have impacted her life and how she practices as a Lactation Consultant.

In the beginning, like many breastfeeding advocates, when she had her first child, she didn't know how to breastfeed and had many difficulties. She dropped in on a local La Leche League meeting and knew she had found a home. Although she felt a connection to the leaders over the next year, it seemed somewhat one-sided, and it wasn't until she went to an international La Leche League conference on her own that she realized she wanted to help others with breastfeeding. She credits this realization more to the atmosphere created by moms and babies than a single inspirational person or experience. She felt that her training was good and encouraging, but that she had trouble feeling an emotional connection. She describes one of her trainers in particular.

"She was the perfect mom, La Leche League Leader, and woman. I mean, I wanted to be her, right down to the way she wore her hair, and how others saw her. However, she was too perfect, there was just <u>no way</u> it was going to happen for me because I can NEVER be like that. I wanted to, badly, but it was impossible- and I never saw her without thinking that."

Ann's second and most influential person came at the lowest point in her life. She was trying to cope with grief after losing a child, attempting to jump start a new career, and had a new set of twin boys at age 47-and couldn't produce enough milk for them. Any one of these scenarios can be paralyzing, if not devastating, but for a new IBCLC, the breastfeeding issues were the final straw.

"She started off as my lactation consultant and would come to my house after working all day, and help me when I knew she was tired. There were evenings when she cried over me, and I cried with her-she was never afraid to show how she felt."

That empathy continued as Ann asked her LC to become her professional mentor. After all of the life challenges, she didn't feel ready to work on her own, but she knew that she still wanted to help nursing mothers. She gained confidence over time, mostly from the verbal feedback from her mentor, rather than the clinical skills she was exposed to. Thinking back, Ann states,

"Whenever I had a difficult patient, she would always say "you get the most difficult and tough cases for a reason!' She made me realize that I wasn't stupid, that I could handle it."

They ended up with a strong emotional connection that lasted long before and after the professional relationship.

"She brought me food when I was a new mom, and I brought her food when she was diagnosed with cancer."

Ann credits both of her mentors for giving her the behavior tools that she uses today. She states that she is never afraid to show her flaws and how she feels. She never wants a mother to believe that she can't relate. She always wants to let others see her compassion.

Preparation Ground Work

Whether preparing to be a mentor or a trainer, you must first look at your own existing constraints in your current role. A learner may pick up on new topics or skills rapidly, but will still require much discussion about observations and rationale. This starts with a basic pencil and paper activity. Some things to consider/questions to ask yourself as a potential mentor are:

Current job requirements:
- What is a typical day for you?
- Are you able to get all of your patients seen effectively or do you leave feeling like you wish you could spend more time on assessment?
- Can you make a list of everything you do, every day? Once a week or monthly items?
- Do you have tasks that you routinely "let go"?
- Do you have any down time? How frequently does that occur?
- Do you have support from your supervisor for mentoring?

Additional roles and responsibilities
- Are you active in other organizations or clubs, such as breastfeeding coalitions? How much time does that require?
- Do you take on special projects, such as health or baby fairs, website updates, and/or World Breastfeeding Week events? Is this something you have help with?
- Do you have unrelated roles that can overlap (small children, church, elder care)?

Practice areas
- Do you have more than one practice area?
- What types of scenarios or learning opportunities are available?

- Is there a mentoring program already in place or will you have to create one?
- What are some ways you can expose your intern to other practice settings?
- Do you have a back-up LC if you are unable to work? Is this someone who can also help with training?

Practice Challenge One:

You are a hospital lactation consultant, working straight eight hour days, Monday-Friday. You typically have about 8-10 patients to round on, and may also have an outpatient consult or two. You are additionally responsible for follow up calls for discharged moms and answering any warm line calls that come during your shift. Every year, you participate in the annual baby fair at the local mall, and you are active in your community breastfeeding coalition. One of the staff nurses has approached you about becoming a lactation consultant, and she wants you to train her.

- *What should your initial response be?*
- *How can you determine if this is something you can take on?*
- *Will you have enough time for this responsibility?*
- *What are some steps you can take to ensure that she obtains a well-rounded education?*

Common Challenges

Mentoring can come with a distinctive set of challenges. The biggest challenge to the seasoned LC who has spent years in practice is to learn how to identify and communicate her practice behaviors. This can be very difficult for the person who practices by instinct because she is no longer stopping to think through why she does the things she does-she just does them. Sometimes this can create a huge communication barrier if she believes she is being clear, but her learner still can't keep up. This difficulty is compounded by the fact that there are two patients instead of one, and during a consult, the primary focus must be on the mother and baby.

To overcome this, it may be helpful for the LC mentor to write out the steps of a consult, using three to five words for each step; first as a rough draft, and then clarified in greater detail. By listing in this format, she can identify the basic process she uses for practice as a foundation. She will then be able to communicate this process to her learner and elaborate; deviating from the steps, as problems are identified. It may even be helpful for her to laminate the final draft of the process for her learner to use as a pocket guide as she progresses through her training.

Another challenge can be identifying when and where mentoring will take place. For the clinical component, three schedules must be coordinated: the mom/baby, mentor, and the learner. In a busy setting, such as a hospital or a WIC clinic, there may be plenty of moms and babies always present, but the mentor and/or learner may be conflicted by other responsibilities that can interfere, but are equally as important. For the PPLC doing exclusive home visits, the challenge is coordinating schedules after down-time, since consults occur without much warning or notice. Of course, the ultimate challenge is coordinating the mentoring opportunity so that it occurs when a baby is ready to eat!

However, when it comes to teachable moments, these can even be found during missed feedings. A full, satisfied baby is a wonderful teaching tool because, in addition to identification of the characteristics of satiety, the mentor can also review physical and developmental signs by assessment, along with gestational age indicators, signs of birth trauma, and other important physical and behavioral characteristics that can be missed when feeding is the focus. If the feeding was poor, post-feed behaviors are even more important to learn because they are often misread by parents and professionals alike.

Personal Inventory

Individuals interested in going beyond being a basic trainer or teacher can start with self-assessment, also known as a personal inventory. This includes making a list of personal and professional strengths and weaknesses. By doing this, a mentor can avoid or at least be aware of common pitfalls, as well as be better prepared for unexpected occurrences. For example, a good mentor must know where and when to set limits in order to avoid personal burnout, particularly if a learner seems needy or doesn't recognize time constraints. A good mentor must also be able to determine when the learner needs autonomy. A mentor should avoid taking over, or explaining too much, because often the best method of learning is by doing. If a mentor is familiar with her own personality traits and tendencies, she can create and identify her own balance between mentoring and her other responsibilities.

There are many types of self-assessment tools that can be easily accessed on the Internet by doing an informal search on Google or other user sites. The simplest tools with only basic definitions of results are free. There is often a fee associated with more complex assessments that come with an in-depth interpretation of results. Which tool to access depends on the interest, motivation, and usage needs of the user. The most common and well known personal assessment is the Myers Briggs Type Indicator (MBTI). This tool is used in a variety of settings, from psychologists for marital counseling to Human Resources staff for job placement criteria. However, it is extremely helpful as a starting or growth tool for anyone mentoring or leading others.

Basically, this and other assessments like it contain a series of questions the user is instructed to answer as honestly as possible, choosing their first response rather than over thinking the questions. The results are interpreted and the emerging profiles consist of strong personality traits that are broken down into usable or recognizable categories. Each trait is defined and compared to its opposite. The individual is assigned one trait in each of four categories, and traits are identified as "this or that." Most people have overlapping characteristics, with one outweighing the other. For the Myers Briggs, the resulting profiles with a very brief description are:

Extraversion (E) or Introversion (I)

Extraversion (**E**)-Generally outgoing, a talker, more comfortable around lots of people as opposed to one-on-one or alone. E's tend to speak before they think because they speak and react to others rapidly.

Introversion (**I**)-The more people that surround the I's, the quieter they get; they are much more comfortable with very small groups or alone. They tend to hold back, wanting to be last to speak, and can even lose the opportunity by waiting too long.

Sensing (S)/Intuition (I)

Sensing (**S**)-The Sensing person tends to take in all of the details, as many as possible. They function in the immediate rather than the "what if's", and like to take a practical, proven approach.

Alternately, the **Intuition** (**I**) person is more of a dreamer, focusing on the potentials and the future rather than the rote activities of today. Often they appear as though they aren't paying attention.

Thinking (T)/Feeling (F)

Thinking (T)-As implied, T's are very cognitive, using strong logic to make analytical, linear types of decisions. This is a direct contrast to the **Feeling (F)** person who operates from "the gut" or the heart, using subjective information, emotions, or personal values for decision making. Even the behaviors are very opposite, T's are often perceived as cold or unfeeling, while F's are considered very emotional and easy to impact.

Judging (J)/Perceiving (P)

The **Judging (J)** personality needs order and structure in their world, is a list maker, and is task oriented. They are good at staying focused until a project or job is complete, sometimes to the exclusion of all else.

The **Perceiving (P)** person is adaptable to changing situations and actually prefers change. They will flow with new ideas or input, but can also be perceived as indecisive or procrastinators.

The benefit of self-assessment in terms of personality is the recognition of how a trainer approaches or reacts to problems and issues, or even ordinary tasks, helping with self-guidance. Large corporations administer personality tests to new hires, particularly in management roles, to better utilize training resources and minimize turnover or training failure. Lactation Consultants are a long way from adopting this process for interns, but the benefits of self-assessment to the mentor affect the learner as well, particularly if the mentor is able to describe how her approach differs from the learner in terms of personality. By emphasizing differences, she can encourage a multi-approach to problem solving.

Practice Challenge Two:

Amy loves that her job as a PPLC is always changing—she never knows when a mama will call for help. Some days she is in her office catching up on her filing, other days she is racing across town trying to fit in several home visits before the end of the work day. Flying by the seat of her pants works well for her personality, and she rarely gets tired of it. She is mentoring an intern who is preparing to take her IBLCE boards in a year.

Her intern shows up every day with a "to see" list and always wants to know exactly what they will be doing. She takes copious notes during every consult and activity, and always asks multiple questions; the questions are often variations of the same thing.

This sometimes makes Amy feel a little irritated because she would rather go with the flow. She also senses that her intern appears frustrated sometimes, and she thinks that it may be because of the lack of daily structure.

- *What personality traits do you think apply to Amy?*
- *What personality traits do you think apply to the intern?*
- *What are some potential problems that can occur if this practice environment and training approach are unchanged?*
- *What are the benefits of this practice approach?*
- *How can Amy identify if there is a problem (or not)?*
- *How can Amy optimize the learning process for her intern?*

Communication

Finally, the emotional aspects of the mentoring relationship should not be undertaken lightly. To mentor requires a full commitment because this is a relationship built on trust. A mentor should not break a relationship unless there is a true life emergency or the relationship has reached a point where learning is no longer possible (see Chapter Eight, Mentoring Breakdown). Communication is a critical part of the trust relationship. A good mentor must be able to articulate assessment findings into a treatment plan with the mother as well as the learner, but both have different needs and starting points. Effective communication is always an ongoing challenge as well as a goal. The mentor is not only role modeling this for patient interactions, but also for future trainee's-particularly if her intern goes on to teach others. A mentor must be able to communicate learning needs, errors, and potential conflict issues in a way that is non-confrontational or critical, but instead creates a guidepost for the learner. In a situation where safety is a concern, communication must be very clear and absolute.

Just as important, a mentor must be able to communicate well *about* her trainee. A mother should always be introduced to the learner and given a brief explanation for the learner's presence. The mother should be informed that she has the option of refusing to have the learner present during her consult. This rarely happens, but it is always a possibility, so the learner should be reassured that it isn't personal if it occurs. Sometimes hospital or organizational staff can be slow to accept a substitute if the mentor is transitioning an intern into unsupervised consults. A mentor who takes the time to create an environment of support can alleviate possible resistance, as well as build confidence in her learner and in the healthcare team.

A Personal Story
Sharon Lilienthal, IBCLC

Shannon Lilienthal started her professional life as a social worker, but after several years of working with families in crisis, she found herself experiencing severe career burnout. To determine a career direction, she explored several resources that involved self testing for personality traits and professional affinities, which led her to seek training in breastfeeding support-unusual because she didn't have a medical background or any children of her own.

She met her mentor while enrolled in a hospital internship program, role shadowing various Lactation Consultants. When recalling her early days with her mentor, she gets choked up describing her experience.

"The best thing about her was how she spoke positively of me to others on the hospital floor. When nurses would ask her for help with a breastfeeding mom, she would encourage the nurse to find me instead, and would also go on to tell them about my strengths and experience working with young low-income mothers. I don't know if she did this with everyone as a training technique, but I do know that it made me feel wonderful, as well as confident. I knew others respected her skills and experience very highly, which made the things she said about me that much more important. I felt that no matter what happened, she had my back. If my mentor believed in me, then they would too because they trusted her opinion."

Shannon's internship led to a full-time position at the hospital. Shannon felt that the hospital staff often viewed her with skepticism because she was young and new to the field. Even after the formal relationship ended, her mentor continued to help her to find the confidence to succeed and played a vital role in helping others on staff see her true talents. She states that she learned a lot clinically from all of the LC's, but that it was the nurturing and professional role modeling of her mentor that created a strong impression and a feeling of empowerment.

This translates into how Shannon trains others, even down to encouraging passionate moms to consider training as a peer counselor to advocate for other moms. She always remembers to give positive words of encouragement.

Chapter 4. Creating the Program

Currently there are a variety of formal and informal mentoring programs available to individuals working toward becoming Lactation Consultants. However, the need or demand appears to be outstripping the number of existing programs or opportunities. In addition, some programs, such as peer counseling through WIC, are only available to a specific type of learner.

Hospital Programs

Hospital mentoring programs are one of the fastest growing and most readily available opportunities for learners. Structured as a formalized teaching/clinical environment, learners are processed into the medical system through routes similar to nursing or other healthcare students. They must have clear urine drug screens, healthcare provider CPR certification, and postpartum depression (PPD) and other screenings. In addition, there is typically an application process including interviews, reference checks, and letters of recommendation. Programs that are successful with the administrators or coordinators take a business approach to the program. This can keep costs down, create staff development opportunities that occur when a program is in process, and create a pool of potential employees within the learners. An active mentoring program can be used as a marketing tool for the organization as well. Hospital programs are typically fee-based, although some of the overhead costs may be absorbed by the organization or by grant or foundation funding.

A Personal Story
Linda Kutner RN, IBCLC
Hospital Lactation Consultant

At Lake Norman Hospital, one intern is accepted per year, although there are multiple Lactation Consultants on staff. In addition to a typical admission process, the hospital requires that only healthcare professionals are accepted into the program. The intern is responsible for her own coursework and has a good deal of input on her learning process as it progresses. She initially role shadows all of the LCs, while learning basic procedures and routines, but her education very quickly becomes hands on. Linda Kutner takes an active role mentoring interns, but she also privately teaches "train the trainer" type courses for mentors.

"They will start off doing weights very early" reports Linda. "Starting weights, ac/pc weights, this will get them comfortable with holding and manipulating the baby."

Linda also describes the difficulty of identifying levels of acuity for teaching interns or other learners.

"In nursing, you start off with giving bed baths, and work your way up from there. In lactation, we can't do it that way. You don't know what you are getting until you walk in that room. Even then, sometimes you don't identify the complicated patients until you are well into the consult."

For this reason, if the intern has been practicing unsupervised, but then wants to take a day to role shadow an LC to learn a different technique or focus on a specific task, she only has to request it. Linda says,

"I don't want her to get done fast. I want her to learn that there are several different approaches for doing it the right way. When she tells me that my way is different from anyone else and that's why she wants to follow me for a day, I feel good that she is comfortable enough to say that and can recognize it."

Linda feels that for a hospital to consider starting an internship program, there must first be a well established lactation support system with full inpatient support (with back up), an outpatient service that is fee-based, "not free," and is fully operational. There must also be a structured training system that can remain in place even with employee turnover.

Hospital mentoring is a great learning opportunity, even without a formal program in place. The difference is that the learners would typically come from within the hospital system. Even in organizations with ideal LC to birth ratios (2.6 FTE's/1000 births, Mannel, 2006), there are not enough hours in the day to fully support all breastfeeding mothers, train staff, run classes, and accomplish all of the other expected tasks. Mentoring others is a great way for the ILC to extend the support line for mothers. One way to do this is by identifying potential team members that already demonstrate an affinity for breastfeeding support. This can come from staff nurses, techs, birth educators, and other allied health professionals. The ILC can mentor individuals over a short term period and gradually create a team of support that function as "extra hands" for her. The goal is not to create additional Lactation Consultants, but rather advance practice helpers that are available to assist moms when she can't.

Practice Challenge Three:

A small community hospital was only able to budget for a part-time, inpatient Lactation Consultant. This meant that she was available to help moms three days a week. The nursing staff identified a need for more support and approached the clinical manager and the ILC to find a solution. As a result, the concept of the breastfeeding support team was created, and six nurses were identified for the team. The ILC worked one-on-one with each team member while both were on shift, and group team meetings were held every two weeks for additional trainings. Team members were also assigned homework for self-directed learning.

At the end of ten months, two team members had dropped out, but an additional member had been added. Their primary responsibilities were assisting mothers who needed extra help with breastfeeding (while they were on shift), making follow-up calls after discharge to answer very basic questions or refer for additional help resources, and facilitate a breastfeeding support group. They also took an active role in new employee orientation to teach basic breastfeeding support.

- *What are the advantages of creating a breastfeeding team?*
- *What are some of the challenges that can occur, both during training and afterward?*

- *Why do you think some of the members dropped out? Could this have been prevented?*
- *How would you identify potential team members?*
- *What are some of the things that you would teach?*

Peer Counseling

Peer counseling can be compared to niche marketing in the business world. As the name implies, a peer counselor is an individual who helps and supports breastfeeding mothers within her own socioeconomic and cultural community. Simply put, the peer counselor has already faced many of the mother's life challenges and can very much identify with the mothers' personal circumstances. The best known peer counseling programs are through WIC, but other programs include La Leche League International, Nursing Mothers Counsel, and BELLAS. In additional, boutique style programs are being created to serve mothers with NICU or special needs babies.

Peer counselors are typically taught lactogenesis and basic breastfeeding support. But the greatest in-depth instruction is on counseling the mothers. The peer counselor role is more of a listener and advisor. During training, emphasis is placed on making appropriate referrals and role boundaries.

A Personal Story
Jan Ellen Brown IBCLC
BELLAS Peer Counseling Program Board of Directors

BELLAS is a unique peer counseling program in Charlotte, North Carolina. Originally part of the WIC program, BELLAS became a self-standing entity with a focus of mother support that began immediately after birth. Peer Counselors routinely visit area hospitals to connect with low-income moms enrolled in the program to initiate contact before feeding problems occur. The PC remains in contact with the mother for the entire duration of her breastfeeding experience. Jan Ellen Brown takes an active role in the program.

"Our peer counselors are the moms themselves; they have walked in the mothers shoes and know what these moms are going through in a way that I don't. They really speak the language."

Jan Ellen means it figuratively and literally. Most of the peer counselors are bi-lingual, and the second language is not just Spanish. To list a few, BELLAS peer counselors communicate in Ukrainian, Chinese, Russian, Korean, and even American Sign Language. The potential counselors are identified from the existing clientele of nursing moms. Structured training lasts approximately eight months, but education continues as an ongoing process when PCs are sent to conferences and workshops to update or increase their skill sets.

"The good that comes of this program benefits both the mom and the peer counselor, and that is ongoing," says Jan Ellen.

"Of course we can identify the benefits of peer-to-mother support, but I can see the changes in the peer counselor herself. This may be her first real job that isn't flipping burgers or cleaning hotel rooms. She is attending meetings and wearing a name tag with a title, you can see her confidence increasing. The best thing is that a whole new world opens up to these ladies. They can go to a community college and become nurse techs, nurses, medical assistants, or they can go on to become Lactation Consultants. This pollinates back to the moms as well, and they want to be peer counselors, too, because they can imagine themselves in that role. It just keeps going."

Peer counselors can be implemented in any healthcare setting. They are not an exclusive function of public health. In fact, a peer counselor can be the bridge of support between the mother and the breastfeeding expert.

Peer counseling can move beyond the traditional mother-to-mother support for a breastfeeding program. In fact, peer support doesn't have to refer to mothers at all, but rather can be breastfeeding professionals, program coordinators, or even organizations.

A Personal Story
Karen Peters MBA, RD, IBCLC
Executive Director, Breastfeeding Task Force of Greater L.A.

The "Birth and Beyond California Project" is a group/peer mentoring project facilitated by the Breastfeeding Task Force of Greater LA and funded by the Public Health Department and the Maternal Child Health discretionary fund. The group is management/administrator focused with members representing 15 area hospitals. The team meets monthly for approximately two hours and discusses ongoing challenges, such as staffing, meeting patient needs, productivity, costs, and so on. Because the members are primarily maternity care managers or directors, the meeting focus is very different from meetings consisting of lactation staff or mother support groups.

According to Karen Peters, although the Breastfeeding Taskforce is the facilitator, the meetings belong to the members.

"We convene at a different host hospital each time, and all are in rotation so each has a turn. There is a common agenda, but they are learning from each other as they share policies, data, and work strategies from their own facilities. The focus of the project is improvement of hospital support for consistency within the community. In addition, it's a support group for managers."

The ultimate goal of the project is to splinter the starting members into regional groups; they are already identifying future service planning areas. More information can be found at the California Public Health Website (listed in the bibliography).

Private Practice Mentoring

There are many private practice LCs who mentor on an ongoing basis, without formal sanction or programs. They often see it as an expansion of their role as a community healthcare professional; particularly since PPLCs often started off as La Leche League Leaders. The lactation consultant in private practice who mentors has a unique opportunity to improve breastfeeding support within her community, as well as identify potential employees or helpers for business expansion.

PPLCs often report that private practice is where their "real learning" began, typically because the patients are clinically complex. Whether the consult takes place in the office or the mother's home, their situation is often very unique and clinical skills must be cutting edge to deal with surprise scenarios. However, before taking this responsibility on, the PPLC must be aware that she could be impacting her business from a variety of aspects. When determining who and when to mentor, she should carefully consider personality, communication style, even where her potential learner wants to practice when the education process is complete. She should then thoroughly interview and communicate with her learner to ensure that this relationship won't negatively affect her business.

The mentoring arrangement is usually fee driven, since the PPLC doesn't have a salary that covers training others. Sometimes the fee is paid for the learner by her employer; other times she pays it herself, like any secondary education course or program. The PPLC can also consider creating a grant-funded program by adding a non-profit arm to her business or by seeking out funding from sources that don't have the 501c categorization as a requirement. However, if the program is covered by a grant, it's usually a good idea for the learner to also invest in her education, either with work time or financially, in order to obtain a full commitment to the relationship. The barter system is a great way for a learner and PPLC to find a solution for teaching reimbursement. In exchange for a specific mentoring plan with predetermined goals, the learner can agree to work a specific number hours as a class instructor, retailer, or as an independent LC once she passes her boards. If she needs specialized training to work her exchange hours, this should not be included in the mentoring agreement or in payment, although it's definitely an added bonus for her education process. This can include anything from running a cash register to teaching a class.

A Personal Experience
An IBCLC

By request, the lactation consultant will remain anonymous. This IBCLC has a dual role as a private practice LC, as well as a part-time employee within a large organization. Like many PPLCs she struggles with earning a viable income with her business. She lives in a moderate-sized town, with a very limited number of five-year-plus IBCLCs. With the exam pathway changes, she has been approached several times in the last year for mentoring opportunities.

"This is always a no-win situation for me. If I refuse to mentor, I appear mean spirited and unwilling to help educate future LCs-and word gets around in this community, as well as the professional one. If I say yes, I have to do this on my own time,

since the organization isn't willing to pay me for anything more than what they hired me to do in a very specific number of hours. I am very part-time, and the rest of my time and energy goes into building my practice."

She states that the individuals who are seeking clinical mentoring are often offended when she brings up the discussion of fees and payment for training, although they have already paid for related course work and class materials through an established academic program. This, in turn, makes her feel frustrated because she feels that training course coordinators should either better prepare the learners for what to expect when seeking clinical experience or else set up contracts with local LCs for the clinical application. The LC fee could be incorporated into the course cost, saving the learner a lot of time and frustration as well.

At this point in time, although she actually likes teaching and mentoring others, she hasn't been able to find a workable solution.

Private practice mentoring contains many variables in addition to the excellent learning opportunities. Because this tends to be less of a formal practice environment, the PPLC needs to develop a structured program before mentoring begins.

Practice Challenge Four:

The personal story, though it has some unique details, contains many realities for PPLCs. Consider the implications from your own viewpoint, experience, and practice area.

- *Do you think that she should mentor others regardless of the issues? Why or why not?*
- *What are some things that she can do to overcome her concerns?*
- *Who could she call on for help with her challenges? Help with the mentoring process?*
- *What can she do to avoid future conflicts?*

Residency Training

At this point in time, there is not an identifiable mentoring program specific to or exclusively for physicians of any practice area. However, the American Academy of Pediatrics has created a breastfeeding education and support program geared toward residents during their training. They state on their website:

> Breastfeeding is best for the health of infants and mothers. As more mothers are choosing to breastfeed, physicians need to be trained to successfully support these mothers. The American Academy of Pediatrics developed this Breastfeeding Residency Curriculum to help residents develop confidence and skills in breastfeeding care. It can be applied to Pediatric, Family Medicine, Preventive Medicine, Internal Medicine, and Obstetric/Gynecologic Residency Programs. The curriculum has been organized based on the Accreditation Council for Graduate Medical Education Core Competencies. Included are goals and objectives, as well as planning, teaching, and evaluation tools, prepared cases and presentations, and suggested resources.

This site contains numerous resources and heavily stresses the importance of the clinical exam case study. These materials can be used as a springboard within any teaching hospital that has an obstetrical and pediatric service. Chances are that there is a lactation program already in place with outpatient services as well, although there may not be a mentoring program established. It would benefit residents of any specialty to initially role shadow, and then complete their clinicals under observation of the IBCLC. Ideally, the residents should be exposed to not only the new postpartum mother and baby in the hospital setting, but also at a birth center, outpatient consult, WIC or public health clinic, and even at a home visit with a PPLC. This will give them a greater understanding of the role of the LC, which will be helpful as they begin their own medical practice, but more importantly, provide a detailed exposure to the more complex lactation cases. Role shadow observations can be single cases, in a few hours over several days, or by rotation and part of the established curriculum.

Chapter 5. Mentoring Tracks

Mentoring can be short- or long-term, depending on the needs of the learner. The ultimate goal is to expose the learner to the practical application of lactation knowledge. In short-term mentoring, hands-on application by the learner is either limited or doesn't occur at all. The goal of long-term or structured mentoring is autonomy for the learner. Because mentoring consists of varied types of relationships, it may be helpful to think of each type as a "mentoring track." The type of mentoring relationship or track is dependent on the programs, the learner, the mentor, and the learning needs.

Observation Opportunities

An observation opportunity is a snapshot view of the LC or trainer in practice. The observation may be a day on the job of one lactation consultation. The observation is deliberately short and typically involves a learner who is considering the field of lactation or someone who wants a better understanding of a particular practice environment or skill. The observation can take place in an office, clinic, home, hospital unit, or patient room. An observation can even take place at a conference, where an IBCLC breaks down the steps of a full consult, with a mother and baby present, to a small group of attendees.

The intent of an observation opportunity is not to teach the full mechanics of lactation or the other aspects of rendering care (interviewing techniques, documentation, assessment), but rather to focus on predetermined specifics or provide a broad overview. Once a general program guideline is established, hours spent in preparation are very limited on the LCs part, since the learner can be given an overview of a consult and the elements of breastfeeding support before the observation. Time should be blocked after a consult for a brief case discussion in order to clarify any questions the learner may have. Learners may spend a couple of hours to a full day on observation, but this should not be extended longer because of the intentional brevity of this role.

Observations provide a multitude of benefits for the giver and receiver. It can serve to highlight an existing lactation program or service, much like a marketing tool: actions speak louder than words. It can educate emerging or new healthcare professionals, such as nursing students or pediatric residents, about the role of the LC as a health resource. It can also provide a "work toward" goal for the individual beginning the process of becoming a professional breastfeeding support person.

Practice Challenge Five:

Many RN programs require that nursing students complete a specific number of hours of observation in a community health setting. A home or clinic-based consult is a great way to expose a future healthcare professional not only to evidence-based breastfeeding support, but also to the importance of breastfeeding itself.

You are the owner of a breastfeeding clinic that provides home and office consultations. In your area, there is a university nursing program, and you would like to offer the students a chance to see a lactation consultation. You also have an LC that is willing to mentor for this project. Now, you just need to get the program rolling.

- *What is the best way to get started? How will you let student nurses know about your program?*
- *What are some of the potential costs that you need to consider?*
- *What do you think some of your challenges will be?*

Role Shadow

A role shadow is where the learner follows the LC for consults, with limited hands-on contact with the mother and baby. Learning tends to be observational, as well as question and answer, with practice documentation, and some self-directed learning. Generally, there is a predetermined number of hours or patients, and the role shadow may also include specific learning needs. For example, the initial agreement may be for 20 clock hours, but the shadowing will take place during outpatient consults only, rather than inpatient support. Role shadowing generally includes lengthy discussion of observations, and generally multiple consults are reviewed.

The LC should plan on approximately one to two hours of mentoring time concurrent with the consult, depending on the practice setting. For example, the LC may typically spend one hour with a mother and baby.

When adding teaching time, including details of assessment during the consult, case discussion, documentation, and addressing questions, total time is at least doubled. The LC will also want to include time spent preparing her learner for the upcoming consult, as well as Q&A afterward as part of the total training time cost. Flexibility with tracking training time spent is up to the individual mentor, although "freebie" time should be carefully monitored and limited. This means lengthy phone calls or informal meetings to discuss cases or answer questions. The role shadow can always be extended if needed.

Practice Challenge Six:

Betty has a peer counselor who is shadowing her for a total of 30 hours while she does home visits. The hours are fee-based, covering time spent with patients, as well as case discussion and other training needs. Initially, Betty felt that the process was going well, her shadow asked lots of questions and was very eager to learn. Betty also enjoyed her company while going from one client home to the next; typically she spends the car time listening to books on tape or thinking over cases. She has gotten to know her shadow on a personal level and often thinks that they could end up as good friends. However, role shadowing is starting to feel very slow and time consuming. Her shadow has started lingering longer and longer to continue the discussion at the end of the shift, and also calls Betty with additional questions. Betty is starting to feel torn. She wants to support her shadow, but it feels like work is overlapping into her private life.

- *What is the real problem in this scenario?*
- *How could Betty have avoided this issue?*
  Now that the problem exists, how can is be addressed?
- *Are there any benefits to keeping the relationship as it currently stands? Any disadvantages?*

Group Mentoring

Group mentoring works well when several people have identical or similar learning needs. Generally, for group mentoring to be effective, there should be at least one facilitator or leader to act as a guide and provide direction. The facilitator should probably have a higher level of knowledge and experience or at least be able to locate resources for additional information if the group gets stuck.

The most common example of group mentoring is the study group - individuals preparing for an exam or performance evaluations. However, group mentoring also works when establishing a new program or system. In healthcare organizations, many mid-level or clinical managers form their own groups for sharing ideas, bed control, discussing budget or productivity problems, and labor topics. Lactation Consultants can use group mentoring as a way to identify organizational or community trends, create new support systems, or just to learn different approaches to a similar problem.

A Personal Story
Diane Weissinger, IBCLC, LLLL
Author, Private Practice Lactation Consultant

Diane Weissinger describes her first experience meeting some of her future mentors at a La Leche League meeting.

"At the first meeting, my first thought was "Oh, ick! Spare me! These people are fanatics and there is more to me than this." But then I went back, weeks later, as a thank you for some telephone help and they still had my nametag! They wanted, and expected, me to come. I just couldn't stop thinking about that."

It took her three and a half years to decide to become a Leader herself.

As Diane has evolved from La Leche League Leader to LC, writer to public speaker, she has found that she is drawn to the group-mentoring concept. When doing telephone support, she would call one or two co-leaders for more opinions or information, then shared all of the responses with the mom to allow her to choose what would work best. She also states,

"LACTNET became my mentor. People posted their questions and always got different answers. This made me feel better because if I didn't know the one right answer, they didn't either. It really is an art and science."

At the same time, she created a smaller online group of breastfeeding advocates, leaders, and LCs for the "trivial or dumb stuff I was too embarrassed to ask on LACTNET." She reports that the smaller group helped bolster her confidence, and though the group has dissolved over the years, she still applies this technique to her other small online groups-although she is now confident enough to post on LACNET as well. When considering why group mentoring can work well, she writes her viewpoint,

"The Queen Mary 2 is a very big ship. Coming into harbor, it can't make small course corrections easily or quickly. Instead, it relies on a fleet of very small tug boats (or I imagine it does), each pushing or tugging in a different direction. Some of them probably push directly against each other at times, and cancel each other out. But remove any one of these small tugboats, and the QM2 will drift off course. And once it starts drifting, it takes a lot of work to get it back on track again, or maybe they even give up and dock at a different pier altogether.

I think of tugboats whenever I hear about political dissent, or "If only everyone thought the way I do," or Lactation Consultants with different styles, or just about anything else in society where variety exists and not everyone thinks it should. If everyone were like me, we wouldn't need locks on our doors, granted. But we'd all be wallowing in paper (piles) that need filing.

Ours is a complex, slow-moving, hard-to-change world, and we're all just tiny, narrow-minded, ineffective little tug boats. But thank goodness for every single one of us! We may push and shove against one another sometimes, but remove any of us, and the course of our cultural Queen Mary could be changed forever."

Group mentoring can take place in a general meeting place, by conference call using the telephone or video conferencing, such as Skype, or online in instant messaging rooms or by listservs. Generally for group mentoring to be effective long term, there needs to be an understanding of general ground rules: respectful communication, confidentiality, and active participation by all members. Group mentoring can consist of employees within an organization, community members; or it can even stretch across states or countries. There should be a clear understanding of who the members are, and newcomers should be invited only after group discussion and agreement.

Group mentoring that is effective often creates an environment of open dialogue; introducing a newcomer without group approval can shut down dialogue and dissipate a group very rapidly.

Practice Challenge Seven:

You have created an online discussion group that consists of local breastfeeding advocates in your community. The purpose of the group is to increase breastfeeding rates in the community, which are very low because of the population. You are the facilitator, and your group members communicate by Yahoo message board. The group has grown rapidly and discussion was initially enthusiastic as community issues were identified and solutions offered. However, you have noticed that posts have dropped considerably, and that one person seems to be doing most of the posting. When going back, you notice that most of her posts consist of solution-based statements that primarily contain statements about her own experience and opinions. You are wondering if the group is getting out of balance or too one-sided.

- *What do you think the problem is?*
  If you were the facilitator, how would you address it?
- *How could it have been avoided?*
- *How will you avoid future problems?*

Internship

An internship is a much more detailed mentoring program, designed to be lengthy, with varied clinical exposure, as well as a focus on additional roles and responsibilities of a lactation consultant. Interns often begin with role shadowing, but this is primarily to gain exposure to procedure. Interns build up to a hands-on learning environment, beginning with weighing babies or taking client histories, then expanding to digital suck assessments. They generally finish their training with consults that are not directly supervised, but rather reviewed with the mentor after completion.

An internship should go well beyond the home or office consult. Interns may also learn how to teach classes, develop telephone communication skills, and even discuss basic business practices, since Lactation Consultants often have to define the financial benefits of their work. In addition, LCs are often called on for assistance with creating policies, training programs, and position statements. Writing skills beyond healthcare documentation are a useful tool for interns to develop.

Because an internship is more complex than most of the other tracks, the duration should also be lengthy. An intern should be prepared to devote at least six months to her training, probably longer based on learning needs and curriculum.

Collaborative Mentoring

Sometimes, one person can't provide a diverse learning environment to meet the learner's needs. In this case, collaborative mentoring may be a viable option. With collaborative mentoring, a learning system is created using different practice settings and situations. A preceptor is identified in each setting and is responsible for the learner while she is there. A supervisory mentor oversees the whole process and is responsible for communicating with both the preceptor and the learner. The supervisory mentor is not an administrator in any form, but rather the point person for the program, like the center of a wheel. She is also the individual who builds the trust relationship with the learner and creates the structure for her training.

Practice Challenge Eight:

A local La Leche League Leader with a non-healthcare background is accepted into a hospital internship program with a goal of taking the IBLCE exam when her internship is complete. She has a sound knowledge of breastfeeding support and communication techniques from her years as a Leader. However, she is very unfamiliar with professional support environments. The hospital is a teaching facility with five LCs, 3000 births, and outpatient services, so she will be exposed to a great variety of situations. However, this is only one area of breastfeeding support.

- *How can the intern gain a broader base of experience?*
- *Is she responsible for this? Should she seek her own solutions?*
  What kinds of observations and experiences should she be exposed to that are not directly lactation-based (but can still impact breastfeeding and the role of the LC)?

Collaborative mentoring most often works within an internship. If a collaborative mentoring program is established, the mentor can reach out to the community resources so that her intern can spend some time in area WIC clinics, pediatric offices, health departments, and in home consultations. In addition, depending on state regulations, it would also be a benefit for an intern to observe a home or birth center delivery, as well as hospital births. Particularly beneficial to observe are high-risk births often found in teaching hospitals.

Imprinting

Ann Conlon-Smith makes the statement, "Maybe you don't have one mentor. Maybe it's all of those women who help us at different points in our life."

Imprinting is a word often used by breastfeeding experts. It is the description used when encouraging early feedings to initiate the breastfeeding relationship. LCs, like Jeanne Rago, use it to describe memories that she considers while describing early mothering influences. Scientists use it when defining an animal's (including humans) innate response to specific stimuli. Imprinting can also be a form of mentoring.

Even those not actively involved in a mentoring relationship can have a big impact on others. For Lactation Consultants, this is a form of imprinting, the very thing we encourage expectant and new mothers to do with their babies. An imprint is an indelible impression or memory. For example, many personal stories of LCs begin with a particular individual who helped them with breastfeeding. This was someone who came in and out of their life very briefly when examined in consideration of the span of a lifetime. However, during this brief encounter, there was an emotional connection that is often remembered by the receiver long after the event.

In Her Words

Stacy D. Kucharczk MSN, RN, CPNP, IBCLC
Pediatric Nurse Practitioner

Here is a small story: The first person who pops into my mind when you mention mentor is an IBCLC who I met at a local lactation conference; the first time I had ever attended. I also attended the pre-conference which was a clinical-skills day. I sat next to this IBCLC and she introduced herself and her colleagues who were there with her. One of the skills station was hand expression of breast milk, with a mom who was demonstrating. I was fascinated; this was before I had children, and although I had worked a lot with breastfeeding mothers, this was something that had not come up. After the mom demonstrated how to do it, they asked if anyone wanted to try (hand expression on the mom). I NEVER in a million years would have had the nerve to do it on my own, but the IBCLC encouraged me to try it, and so I did. I was later able to put this skill to use when I had a mama come in terribly engorged and I helped her to hand express to comfort. Although this seems like such a simple act of encouragement that really isn't noteworthy, I think it epitomizes the lactation community as a whole: individuals who enjoy sharing their knowledge and welcoming newbies into their world.

If the LC is unable or uninterested in formal mentoring, she can still help and make a difference to those around her. Lactation Consultants have the opportunity to turn "imprint" into an action verb. Much like the brand name Google has become "googling" when referring to an Internet search, we can become Imprinters, not only for the mothers we reach out to, but just by offering small helps through advice or words of wisdom and encouragement to each other.

Chapter 6. Identifying a Learner

Breastfeeding advocates come from a variety of backgrounds and can be male or female, although females are the huge majority in this field. Advocates often have a passion for breastfeeding that starts from personal experience as a new mother, patient interaction, or even a researcher fascinated with the amazing health benefits of human milk. The knowledge base may be as basic as a high school education up to a full PhD in science. The learner may be a school teacher or a pediatrician. Regardless, identifying a mentoring candidate requires more than just saying yes during a phone call. Dr Ruth Lawrence states,

"Individuals who help mothers' breastfeed should be screened, educated, and trained as well. They should have the following special abilities:

- To *listen*

- To avoid judgment

- To understand other lifestyles

- To admit it when they do not know

- To seek appropriate help from professionals

- To recognize incompatibility in a given relationship

  (Lawrence, 1999)."

How It Begins

Traditionally, an in-depth mentoring relationship, such as an internship, begins when both parties are at least acquaintances. However, as the field of lactation continues to grow at a rapid rate, this may not always be the case. Regardless, there has to be some sort of emotional connection for mentoring to truly be effective. If the mentoring program is large and learners are coming in as strangers, it's better to begin with a role shadow or some sort of brief trial period with a clear end point, before moving forward. This protects both the mentor and the learner from wasting time and resources, as well as preventing negative fall-out if there isn't a good fit.

Practice Challenge Nine

You receive a phone call from a mom you have helped in the past. She loved her breastfeeding experience and tells you she spends a lot of time helping and supporting her friends. She knows that you teach others because you had an intern with you when you saw her. She says,

> *I am not a nurse, but I really want to be a lactation consultant anyway. Can you take me on? I am willing to do anything you say and will clean pumps and answer your phone or give you free labor while you are training me.*

- *How should you initially respond?*
- *How can you determine whether or not to train her?*
- *What is the best way to encourage her without promising something that you can't deliver?*

The Interview

All candidates should be interviewed, regardless of experience, practice setting, or mentoring pathways. If the mentoring is done by observation opportunity, a brief telephone interview and discussion to identify learning needs, as well as state the rules and expectations for the learner will suffice. However, for a more in-depth track, the interview should really be done in person; if that is impossible, a video conference is a less than desirable second choice. Written, electronic, or telephone instruction should be given to the candidate regarding the interview and should include any document requests, such as resume, personal and professional references, and/or copies of certification. The candidate should be told approximately how long the interview will last and the topics to be discussed. She should be encouraged to consider her own questions for you, which she can write down if needed.

Even if you are considering mentoring someone you know well, an interview sets the tone for a new aspect of the relationship, as well as identifies expectations on both sides. Before the interview, ask the candidate to prepare ahead by considering and answering some basic questions, and instruct her to write her answers down.

1. What are your personal strengths?

2. What are your personal weaknesses?
3. What are your professional strengths?
4. What are your professional weaknesses?
5. What are you hoping to gain from this relationship?
6. What are your immediate and long-term goals?

At the beginning of the interview, consider how the candidate presents herself. Appearance alone is not an indicator of work quality, but definitely can impact decision making. For example, a candidate who presents herself in too-tight, revealing clothing already presents a problem that needs to be addressed if a mentorship is offered. Long fingernails, no matter how beautifully polished, present a safety and hygiene risk for a healthcare professional. These types of elements must be taken into account.

There are specific questions that, by law, must be avoided during an interview; typically, these focus on the personal life or health history of the interviewee. However, in many cases, if the candidate herself brings up the subject of her children, you can ask her to elaborate on her statements. If you are uncertain about interviewing topics, you can contact your Human Resources department or state Department of Labor.

The interview should begin with the candidate work and education history. You can and should take notes directly on the resume or on paper that you can attach later. It is helpful to identify what she liked and didn't like about past jobs, as well as any formal education. This will give you a feel for learning needs, how she learns, and what appeals to her. It will also give you an idea about how well she communicates her thoughts and impressions, and even her level of self confidence. This discussion should naturally lead into her answers for the preparation questions that you requested in advance. Again, it is helpful to take notes during the interview, but your attention should be on her, not your paper.

At least half of the interview should focus on expectations, both hers and yours. In addition, the mentor should switch roles and allow the candidate to do the interview, asking her own questions to get a feel for the relationship, since a two-way trust must develop for effective mentoring. The interviewer should be prepared to discuss her own background, as well as strengths and weakness. Sometimes this discussion makes an individual more approachable. This can also allow for realistic expectations of you and the relationship, and may open the door for further communication if she is having learning or communication difficulties. The types of questions she asks you will give you a better idea of her personality and communication styles.

The interview should finish with a basic overview of the mentoring pathway or program, with intention to further discuss the learning plan in greater detail if the candidate is offered a position. The discussion should include anticipated costs and related fees, as well as professional expectations of the learner. The interview should always end by asking for further questions, and thanking the candidate for their honesty and time. You should tell the candidate when and how she can expect to receive your decision, and you must follow through on this exactly. If there is an unexpected delay in decision making, professional courtesy obligates you to communicate this, as well as determine a new deadline.

Making the Decision

An added consideration for acceptance into a program is how the candidate follows up the interview. A very professional response is a written, or at the very least, emailed thank you note from the candidate within three to four days of the interview, that also contains a restated interest in the program or opportunity. This speaks volumes about professionalism.

When considering a candidate, the overall concern should be that there is a connection with the individual. That means the candidate doesn't have to necessarily communicate the same interests or background, but rather there should be an identifiable similarity. Sometimes this is unexpected. The candidate may be your total opposite. But when she talks about the joy she gets seeing a new mother bond with her baby, you recognize your words coming out of her mouth. It may be as subtle as identifying a work ethic. This is hard to define because it is often a feeling or a spark. However, it can't be forced, so if your instincts are telling you it's not a good fit, then it probably won't be--even with ideal intentions.

It's probably helpful, when interviewing multiple candidates for limited positions, or even one position, to list all of the pros and cons of each, then destroy the list once the decision is made. In addition, if there are several positions and preceptors or trainers are used, it's probably a good idea for at least one other person to interview the candidate. The two of you should compare impressions and considerations when making the final decision.

Chapter 7. Getting Started

Once the decision has been made to proceed with mentoring a specific candidate, the mentor and her learner should again meet to establish track guidelines. This will generally take longer than the interview and also involves basic procedural activities. Depending on the program, before the first meeting, the learner may need to complete some tasks, such as taking a CPR class, submitting healthcare screening documents, obtaining a uniform, and so on. These requirements should be issued in writing, typically when accompanied by an offer of mentorship. In a less-formal mentoring environment, expectations that need to be met in advance can be stated by phone.

Creating the Individualized Track

During the initial meeting, the mentor should begin by outlining the learning process. Depending on the track, this may be very detailed, or it may be an overview. For example, the learner who has been accepted for role shadowing during inpatient hospital consults will only need some basic instructions to start. This would include where to present herself, what to do before coming to shadow, what behaviors are expected from her, what she will see and do, where her resources are, and an anticipated learning plan. It is very helpful for both the learner and the mentor to create a chart or some sort of record, not only to track learning needs, but also for ongoing evaluation and to confirm mastery.

Finally, there should be a written agreement, such as a mentoring contract, that is reviewed and signed by both the learner and the mentor, with a finalized copy given to both, and a third copy kept on file if the program is affiliated with an organization. The contract can be as basic as an outline of expectations and program requirements, or it can be a formal legal document with a non-compete clause, fee structure, and processes followed if the mentorship is discontinued. It's a good idea to have any contract reviewed by an attorney who can identify needs that you may not have considered, or statements that should be clarified or removed. If the contract is basic, once reviewed it can generally be adapted to any mentoring track or situation.

As the track progresses, new learning needs and opportunities are invariably identified, so the education plan must have some flexibility. However, it is the responsibility of the mentor to ensure that the learner doesn't stray too far from the original plan, particularly during the shorter tracks with a limited learning time. Some of the learner's education must be self-directed. The mentor can accomplish this by assigning homework or using unexpected case presentations or complications as research suggestions for the learner.

Education of the Adult Learner

The learner may not realize what she doesn't know until the mentoring relationship is already established. Often, once this occurs, the learner can feel overwhelmed and intimidated, and may be afraid to communicate learning needs. She may also start off with the impression that her academic knowledge or past experience is adequate; only to later discover that she still has much to learn before she is prepared to practice.

"I decided to sit for the very first exam in 1985. I figured hey, I had been a La Leche League Leader for 15 years, I surely knew what I was doing. I bought the Lawrence book Breastfeeding: A Guide for the Medical Profession *to prepare. Then I cried through the first four chapters because I didn't know anything! I passed the exam, so it all turned out ok, but I have never forgotten that feeling."*

Kay Hoover MEd, IBCLC

Mentoring a learner can be very similar to teaching a prenatal class to a new mother. There are lots of different types of learning environments, along with a variety of methodologies. The three main areas of adult learning are cognitive (thought processing), psychomotor (behaviors using action), and affective (involving feelings and emotion). In addition, many people consider themselves visual (sight), auditory (hearing), or kinesthetic (hands-on) learners. Any good class involves many types of learning platforms. It is, therefore, critical to use a variety of teaching methods to get the point across during mentoring as well.

Methodologies, or how to teach a particular subject or class, can include role playing, using audio/visuals, discussion, demonstration, and game playing to name a few. For example, the benefits of breastfeeding in a prenatal class can be addressed strictly by lecture, but how much will the audience retain? This subject contains a large volume of research-based information that can easily overwhelm "the message," why mom should breastfeed. Alternatively, this information can be more effectively communicated through discussion or a game involving visuals. The participants can teach each other or themselves, and with the instructor as a facilitator, questions can be addressed on the spot and myths can be clarified. This same format can be used for teaching an intern about palate formation. The mentor can start with a discussion about various types and assessment techniques. The learner uses Q&A after consults to further identify specific types. Finally, the mentor can create a game, using pictures of different palates for the learner to identify types. This helps to evaluate the process and confirm mastery of a topic.

An example of meeting a psychomotor learning need is teaching breastfeeding positions. Because of the importance of the topic, the information can be communicated first in discussion format, using video or pictures to illustrate your statements. Learning is reinforced by providing a doll for the learner to practice different feeding positions for nursing. Finally, the learner can teach an expectant mother, and then a new mother, positioning. This is will further educate her on the different learning needs of those she will encounter once her own track is complete.

There is an old saying used in many education settings: "See one, do one, teach one." However, when mentoring breastfeeding advocates, it may be more appropriate to say, "See many, do lots, then teach with help before soloing."

Ongoing Assessment and Evaluation

To determine effective teaching and learning in any setting or relationship, there must be ongoing assessment and evaluation. This can be as simple as question and answer, soliciting feedback, written testing, performance testing, case presentations, or role playing. In fact, a broad variety of these examples and more should be used in order to measure learning.

Most important, the learner herself should be solicited and encouraged to input and evaluate her progress. Doing so will create a self-advocate within the learner, so that she assumes an active role in her own education. This will need to continue once she finishes her mentorship, so it's best to foster this sense early and often.

Chapter 8. Mentoring Breakdown

Not all mentoring relationships turn out well. Sometimes they end prematurely. On rare occasions, they end badly. This doesn't mean that there isn't a benefit to an unexpected outcome; rather the opposite. Surprises allow the mentor to examine her teaching styles, and interviewing and communication techniques. It also allows for program evaluation, hopefully by both the mentor and the learner.

The Stalled Relationship

Sometimes the mentoring relationship stalls due to unexpected life changes, personality conflicts, or a change in goals. It is the responsibility of both the mentor and learner to identify a solution for improvement, but the mentor may need to articulate the problem first. A learner may feel uncertain or even afraid to bring up an issue for fear of causing offense. She may even be unable to identify the issue.

Often times, a stall is first identified by a feeling that things aren't going well or proceeding in an anticipated direction. Maybe the learner is slow to pick up concepts or doesn't respond or demonstrate an increase in skills or knowledge. If this is occurring, the mentor must first determine what the problems might be, or at the very least, her own concerns about the process. She should identify specific examples, rather than subjective feelings and emotions. Once she is clear on her own viewpoints and issues, she should then discuss these with her learner. The mentor should create a quiet neutral zone for this discussion whenever possible, such as a library or a cafeteria or coffee shop during non-busy hours.

Generally, a stalled relationship occurs for one of two main reasons: ineffective teaching or a change in learning desires. The mentor may not be communicating effectively or clearly, and as a result, the learner is frustrated, confused, or has lost focus. Alternately, the learner may have changed her mind about the process or the goal. For example, her original goal may have been to become a peer counselor, but now that she has been through the first two of six months training, she may have decided that this is not a strong enough interest after all. By initiating the discussion in a non-confrontational way, this can allow the learner to safely communicate her own impressions and feelings.

Sometimes, simply changing the learning environment can make a difference. For example, if the practice area isn't allowing the learner exposure to different approaches to a common problem, the mentor can call on a community partner for help. The pediatric office LC who is teaching her learner about support of the low-income mom can call on the local WIC office for either role shadowing or for her learner to attend a prenatal class with participants. The mentor can still oversee her learning objectives, but the clinical and practice exposure is directly supervised by someone else.

If the learner has changed her mind about the program, help her identify if a different environment, track, or mentor would benefit her, or if she no longer wants to move forward in this direction at all. This is not personal and has nothing to do with the mentor, and it's to the learner's credit that she recognizes this, rather than becoming an indifferent or poor lactation professional.

Evidence-Based and Safe Practice

Sometimes the issue isn't insufficient clinical exposure, but rather safety concerns. A common example is the fine line between empathy and sharing, and presenting subjective experience as implied fact. As learners grow more comfortable with client interaction, they sometimes speak freely and communicate personal opinions. The mentor may observe that the intern is giving advice based on personal experience. An example of this as a safety issue would be the intern who tells new mothers in a prenatal class that she has seen a lot of babies who only need to feed at one breast per feeding, and that the mother can pump the other side and store for future use. Giving such individualized advice before breastfeeding is even initiated, not to mention without knowing the mother's health (or surgical) history could really create a big problem very quickly. The mentor has a responsibility to address potential safety issues immediately during the class, and again privately with the intern.

Step One. The mentor should first correct any misinformation, implied or actual, that was given by the learner to the receiver. This may be to a mother directly or a class. It is not necessary or professional to publicly chastise the learner, and doing so will reduce the clarity and efficacy of the message. Instead, the mentor should correct the error diplomatically, but in no uncertain terms as to the correct information, and leave it at that.

Step Two. The mentor should immediately, or as soon as possible, ask the learner for her own explanation and viewpoint, including why and how the information was delivered.

Step Three. The mentor should explain the rationale behind the need for correction, as well as give the information in correct form. This is not "shame and blame," but more of a teacher-student approach. If they don't make errors, how will they learn?

In general, safety concerns can be addressed and resolved fairly quickly by an alert mentor. It is tempting to overlook small issues that don't appear to adversely affect a client, but the issue will repeat if unchecked or uncorrected. Many learners will present personal experience as fact once or twice, but it shouldn't go beyond that. Corrective reinforcement should resolve this. However, if a pattern starts to emerge, no matter how subtle, the mentor will need to keep a written record of any issues, as well as how they were addressed. If the safety concern goes beyond simple misinformation, the corrective measures may need to be more serious and may include the decision to end the mentorship. This is not stated to the learner as a threat, but rather a consequence of actions.

Practice Challenge Ten:

Cathy has an intern who is very outgoing and loves her work with new mothers. She has just started unsupervised consults, so Cathy calls the mothers at home for follow-up once she has reviewed her intern's consult notes. When she calls the third mom, who was seen with a one- month-old for an intake assessment, she is told,

"I am just confused about one thing. My baby is spitting up a lot, so Cathy told me to give her some rice cereal after nursing to help keep her milk down. I thought I wasn't supposed to do this until the baby is older."

- *What should Cathy do first?*
  How can she approach this with her intern?
- *Is this a safety issue?*
- *How can this be prevented in the future?*

Precipitated Endings

Sometimes the mentoring agreement ends prematurely because of unexpected reasons. The intern may be moving, get pregnant, experience a financial downturn, have a death in the family, or some other life interruption that is totally beyond anyone's control. Good can come from an unexpected change; perhaps the mentor can help her intern find a program in her new city or put the internship on hold until life settles down. Even if the mentorship stops, the knowledge acquired by the learner doesn't disappear. If her situation allows, she can teach prenatal classes or run a support group or function as a breastfeeding helper. One intern who couldn't complete the program, went on to work as an LC assistant, answering basic phone call questions, doing bra fittings, and teaching baby care classes. Because of her training, she is very good at reassuring new mothers, but also knows exactly when to refer for a higher level of care. Another intern just couldn't pick up on the medical knowledge needed to be a lactation consultant. However, her empathy for mothers, nurturing personality, and common-sense breastfeeding support made her an excellent home helper for new mamas.

Sometimes, in spite of trying alternate options, the mentoring relationship fails. This can occasionally create a lot of negative feelings between the mentor and learner. Clear communication, with concrete examples, can alleviate some of the negative fall out so that the ended relationship doesn't come as a surprise. For process improvement, there should be an exit interview with the mentor, stressing that this is not a negative consequence, but rather an open dialogue. If this is not possible, the exit can be completed by a trusted third party who can communicate the results to the mentor. Although this scenario can be very discouraging, it is actually a good thing in terms of change and growth. Failure is as important as success in terms of learning and can reinforce positives.

Early endings can leave a mentor with a sense of loss and even sadness. This is not unexpected. A good mentor tends to pour herself into a learner, and this comes with an emotional price tag. Talking out feelings and emotions can help a mentor move on to the next learner. It may help the mentor to focus on past successes and to make contact with individuals who successfully completed the mentoring program in the past. Their continued triumphs and growth can be a source of validation and even comfort. In addition, an unexpected outcome can allow a mentor to identify program flaws, or even change needs for future learners.

Chapter 9. Moving On

The mentor and the learner should both identify when the formal mentoring relationship should end, although mentoring often continues informally well beyond this time frame. Often, when there is a mutual trust accompanied by frequent effective communication, separation is a more gradual process--particularly if there will be a shared work environment. However, there needs to be a moving on or a finish point in order for the learner to develop true autonomy and independence. Sometimes the mentor needs to push the learner a little in order for this to occur. By this stage, the mentor will have a good feel for this personality type.

If the learner has completed a short track and the initial connection was strengthened, it may be a good idea for the mentor to encourage an extended track or an internship, if available. This can be a future consideration, rather than an immediate transition.

Many mentors will write letters of recommendation, create a resume, or offer professional career counseling or recommendations to formally mark the end of a mentorship. Others will treat the learner to dinner or have a small "last day" celebration. When complete, it's important for the mentor to file all paperwork and records for review if needed in the future. It's also a good idea for the mentor to have a break in time before taking on a new learner. Sometimes the end of a mentoring relationship brings a recognition of mental and physical fatigue, so the length of the break is very dependent on the individual.

Regardless, the mentor should take the time to consider the benefits and rewards of this and other mentoring relationships, and she should enjoy them while she relaxes.

Glossary of Terms

These terms are used throughout the book, and are briefly defined as they are used within the context of mentoring breastfeeding professionals.

IBCLC/LC: International Board Certified Lactation Consultant, Lactation Consultant

IBLCE: International Board of Lactation Consultant Examiners

ILC: Inpatient Lactation Consultant; hospital or birth-center setting

Imprinting: Creating an indelible impression or memory. The LC who is an **Imprinter** is practicing an informal, but still very important, form of mentoring.

Intern: A learner in a longer term mentoring track that is hands-on and involves more that just lactation consultations.

Observation opportunity: A brief "snap shot" look at a practice or a consult. It generally lasts several hours, up to a half day.

OLC: Outpatient or Office Lactation Consultant; may be hospital, breastfeeding clinic, pediatric, family practice, or obstetrical office setting.

Peer counselor/PC: An individual who is typically of the same socioeconomic or cultural environment as the individual she is assisting. May also include worksite similarities.

Preceptor: Single training used in one-to-one learning; generally considered an expert or advance-practice level instructor. May evolve into a mentor.

PPLC: Private Practice Lactation Consultant; self-employed LC who may practice in her own office or in the clients' home.

Mentoring Tracks: Descriptive term used to describe a specific collection of mentoring relationships.

Resident: Typically used when describing physicians in clinical training, although residency programs are not limited to the practice of medicine. A **residency** is similar to an internship, although it lasts for several years.

Role shadow: A role shadow is a short time frame, typically focused on observation of breastfeeding consults with very limited hands on learning. A **Shadow** refers to the learner who follows and observes the experienced LC.

Trainee: The learner, typically in a group or less individualized learning environment.

Suggested Library for Mentors

The titles below are intended as a starting point for a mentoring library to be used by both mentors and learners. The list is subject to change, dependent on personal preferences and needs.

Professional Textbooks

- *Breastfeeding: A Guide for Medical Professionals,* Ruth Lawrence
- *Breastfeeding After Breast and Nipple Procedures: A Guide for Healthcare Professionals,* Diana West and Elliot Hirsch
- *Breastfeeding and Human Lactation,* Jan Riordan and Karen Wambach
- *Breastfeeding Answers Made Simple,* Nancy Mohrbacher
- *The Breastfeeding Atlas,* Kay Hoover and Barbara Wilson-Clay
- *Clinical Therapy in Breastfeeding Patients,* Thomas Hale and Pamela Berens
- *Core Curriculum for Lactation Consultant Practice,* Rebecca Mannel, Patricia J. Martens, and Marsha Walker
- *History and Assessment: It's All In The Details,* Denise Altman
- *Maternal and Infant Assessment for Breastfeeding and Human Lactation,* Karin Cadwell
- *Medications and Mothers Milk,* Thomas Hale
- *Nursing Mothers Herbal (The),* Sheila Humphries
- *Selecting and Using Breastfeeding Tools,* Catherine Watson-Genna
- *Supporting Sucking Skills,* Catherine Watson-Genna
- *Clinical Experience in Lactation: A Blueprint for Internship,* Linda Kutner and Jan Barger

Parenting Books

It is important for LCs to be able to recommend quality resources for parents and to know what parents are reading, so the titles below are also good for a mentoring library.

- *Breastfeeding: A Parents Guide,* Amy Spangler
- *Breastfeeding Made Simple,* Nancy Mohrbacher and Kathleen Kendall-Tackett

- *Breastfeeding Café*, Pamela Behrman
- *Happiest Baby on the Block (The)*, Harvey Karp
- *No-Cry Sleep Solution: Gentle Ways to Get Your Baby to Sleep Through the Night* (The), Elizabeth Pantley
- *Breastfeeding Mothers Guide to Making More Milk(The)*, Diana West and Lisa Marasco
- *Mothering Multiples*, Karen Gromada
- *Nursing Mothers' Companion*, Kathleen Huggins
- *Nursing Mother, Working Mother*, Gail Pryor and Kathleen Huggins
- *Womanly Art of Breastfeeding (The)*, La Leche League International
- *25 Things Every Nursing Mother Needs to Know*, Jan Ellen Brown and Kathleen Huggins

Finally, LCs are aware that there are poor, or even potentially dangerous, books for parents. These should be included in a mentoring library to teach specific content when mentoring. If purchasing used books from a garage sale or consignment store, the author and publisher will not receive any income (royalties) from this sale. Purchasing a used book is also better than creating activity on the book at the local library.

- *On Becoming Babywise*, Gary Ezzo
- *The Baby Whisperer*, Tracy Hogg

Additional Books or Resources

_____
_____
_____
_____
_____
_____
_____
_____
_____
_____
_____
_____
_____
_____
_____
_____
_____
_____
_____

Bibliography

Books

Allred, A. (2000). *Passion rules! Inspiring women in business.* Oregon: Oasis Press.

Blanchard, K., & Miller, M. (2004). *The secret: What great leaders know.* San Francisco: Berrett-Koehler Publishers, Inc.

Flanders, J. (2004). *Inside the Victorian home: A portrait of domestic life in Victorian England.* New York: W.W. Norton and Co.

Herriot, J. (1982). *The best of James Herriot: Favorite memories of a country vet.* New York: St. Martins Press.

Jeruchim, J., & Shapiro, P. (1992). *Women, mentors, and success.* New York: Fawcett Columbine.

Kozier, B., Erb, G., Berman, A., & Snyder, S. J. (2008). *Fundamentals of nursing: Concepts, process, and practice.* Upper Saddle River, NJ: Prentice Hall.

Lauwrence, R., & Lawrence, R. (1999). *Breastfeeding: A guide for the medical profession.* St. Louis, MO: Mosby.

Riordan, J., & Wambach, K. (2010). *Breastfeeding and human lactation.* Sudbury, MA: Jones and Bartlett.

Shealy, K. (2005). *The CDC guide to breastfeeding interventions.* Atlanta, GA: US Dept of Health and Human Services.

Articles

Finley, F., & Kennedy, M. (2007). Mentoring junior healthcare administrators: A description of mentoring practices in 127 U.S. hospitals. *Journal of Healthcare Management, 52*(4), 260-269.

Galea, C. (2006).The ultimate motivation guide: Yourself. *Sales and Marketing Management, March,* 24-25.

Lauwers, J. (2007) Mentoring and precepting Lactation Consultants. *Journal of Human Lactation, 23*(1), 10-11.

Mannel, R., & Mannel, R.S. (2006). Staffing for hospital lactation programs: Recommendations from a tertiary care teaching hospital. *Journal of Human Lactation, 22*(4), 409-417.

McVeigh, H. et al. (2009). A framework for mentor support in community placements. *Nursing Standard, 23*(45), 35-41.

Miller, M. (2006). Developing an effective mentoring program. *EMA Management,* March, 14-15.

Pittenger, K., & Heiman, B. (2000). Building effective mentoring relationships. *Review of Business, Summer,* 38-42.

Taylor, C. (2009). Mutually supportive. *Nursing Standard, 24*(1), 61.

Websites

American Academy of Pediatrics. (2009). *Breastfeeding residency curriculum.* Retrieved March 2010 from http://www.aap.org/breastfeeding/curriculum/.

Association of Teachers of Maternal Child Health. (2009). *MCH leadership competencies: Self-reflection.* Retrieved January 2010 from http://leadership.mchtraining.net/?page_id=114.

California Department of Public Health (2010) *Birth and beyond California: Hospital training & quality improvement project.* Retrieved March 26, 2010 from *http://www.cdph.ca.gov/HealthInfo/healthyliving/childfamily/Pages/BirthandBeyond CaliforniaDescription.aspx.*

International Board of Lactation Consultant Examiners. (2010). *Clinical competencies for IBCLC practice.* Retrieved January 2010 from www.iblce.org.

International Board of Lactation Consultant Examiners. (2010). *Pathway three guide.* Retrieved January 2010 from www.iblce.org.

La Leche League International. (2009). *A brief history of La Leche League International.* Retrieved January 2010 from http://www.llli.org/LLLIhistory.html?m=1,0,0.

Merriam-Webster. (2010). Definitions and alternates for "mentor." Retrieved March 2010 from http://www.merriam-webster.com/.

National Academies Press/Food and Nutrition Board. (2004). *Infant formula: Evaluating the safety of new ingredients. Background.* Retrieved March 2010 from http://books.nap.edu/openbook.php?isbn=0309091500&page=42

National Library of Medicine/National Institute of Health. (2010). *A history of medicine*. Retrieved February 2010 from http://www.nlm.nih.gov/hmd/index. html.

Oliver, L. (2010). *The Food Timeline FAQs: baby food & A short survey of manufactured baby foods through time*. Retrieved March 2010 from http://www.foodtimeline. org/foodbaby.html.

Martin, R., & Hixxson, J. (2009). *Personality and the team -Value the person*. Retrieved March 2010) from www.teambuildinginc.com/article_mbti.htm.

Personal Interviews

Ann Conlon-Smith, Jan 12, 2010

Catherine Watson Genna, personal email communication, Jan 22, 2010

Cindi Freeman, Jan 13, 2010

Diane Weissinger, Feb 2, 2010, personal email March 4, 2010

Elizabeth Brooks, March 6, 2010

Jan Ellen Brown, December 10, 2009, March 21, 2010

Jeanne Rago, personal email communication

Karen Peters, March 18, 2010

Kathy Mirra, Feb 27, 2010

Kay Hoover, Feb 27, 2010

Larry Garver, March 14, 2010

Linda Kutner, March 19, 2010

Linda Smith, Feb 27-28, 2010, personal email communication March 14, 2010

Roberta Graham de Escobedo, Jan 13, 2010

Sharon Lilean, Jan. 22, 2010

Stacy D. Kucharczk, personal email communication February 10, 2010

Sylvia Boyd, PT, IBCLC, CST, Feb 2, 2010

Ted DuBose, March 10, 2010

Other

Utter, A. (2009). *Professional education network*. ILCA Conference. PowerPoint presentation.

Author Bio

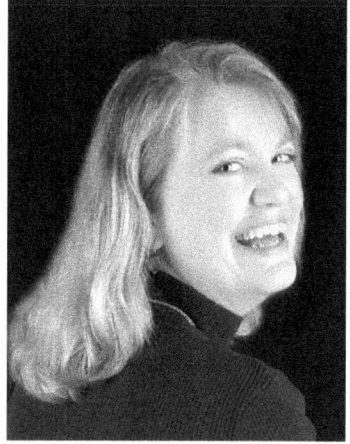

Denise Altman RN, IBCLC, LCCE

Denise Altman is a private practice lactation consultant and nurse educator. She currently owns and operates *All The Best* in Columbia, South Carolina. Prior to that, she has worked in a variety of roles in the healthcare system from staff nurse to clinical educator.

Denise is also a freelance writer, with numerous articles for parents and healthcare professionals in print, in addition to her first book, *History and Assessment: It's All in the Details.* She is a professional speaker who enjoys presenting at both small local venues and international conferences. On a personal note, Denise is the mother of three children.

www.ingramcontent.com/pod-product-compliance
Lightning Source LLC
Chambersburg PA
CBHW070916280326
41934CB00008B/1751